I0710943

<u>REDUCE STRESS!</u>

a cognitive approach

<u>98 Negative Thoughts We Commonly Think, and How to Turn Them Around!</u>

<u>*aka "First World Problems"*</u>

Exercises for your brain

by
Pam Connolly, M.S. Physical Education,
Sport Psychology emphasis and
E. MotionL, N.R.G

1

<u>**Dedication:**</u>

I am dedicating this book to my late mother who we just unexpectedly lost at the end of 2017. Many positive memories and lessons learned flooded my brain, along with the grief I was experiencing. This is a time wherein my objective thoughts met irrational thinking. I didn't know what to say or do one from one moment to the next in the days that followed this shocking news. However, her amazing example of my favorite, personal quote, "focus on the positives in all situations," helped me to look on the bright side sooner than later and carry on with my perceived purpose. She was able to take any negative situation and turn it into a positive, much like what you will do in this book.

I love you mom, and you will be greatly missed.

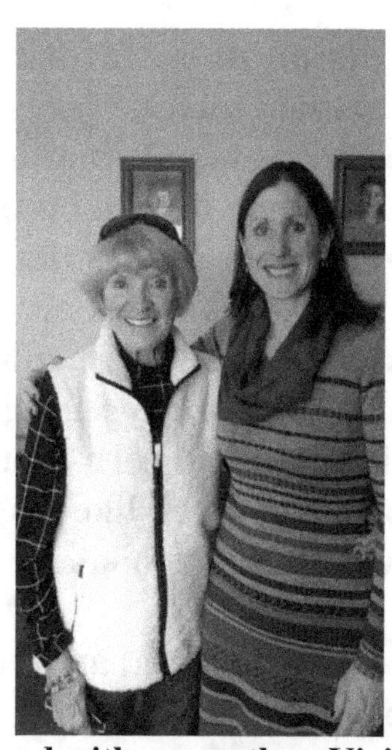

**Pictured with my mother, Vivian G.
Stephens
8-26-39 to 12-27-17**

Introduction:

For years, I have been in the practice of writing down 4-5 things that I am grateful for each day, challenging myself to find different things every day. Practicing what I preach, I was even able to find 5 things to be grateful for on the day my mother passed away. I think that practice, coupled with the following exercise, really helps keep a person grounded and in touch with reality. We may not like or understand our situation, but accepting it is the first step to better manage our stress.

In the late 90's, I earned a certification in Stress Management through the American Association of Lifestyle Counselors. I thought it was a great supplement to my Masters Degree in Physical Education, with a Sport Psychology emphasis that I earned in 1993. One of the topics we learned about focused on our thoughts. Research shows that of all the thoughts we think throughout the day, about half are negative about people, things, or situations. Unfortunately, when we think negative thoughts, our stress level tends to rise. The good news is that we are in charge of the way we think! While it may seem like our thoughts come to us automatically, they are the result of ingrained thoughts or experienced thinking. As soon as we become aware of a thought, we have the choice to continue to think that thought and even act, or, re-think that thought. If the thought is negative, ineffective, and/or unhealthy, we can think a different thought about the situation to lead to a more positive outcome, regardless of whether we act on that positive thought. Furthermore, you can think a different, more healthful thought even if you don't believe it at the time! Cognitive dissonance means that the mind and body do not like to be at odds. Think how you want to be, and you'll eventually become! Get your mind and body on the same page. You can always control your attitude about a situation, even if you can't change the situation itself.

I have used the following exercise with numerous students in Stress Management and Relaxation classes I have taught, as well as in various presentations.

REDUCING STRESS...ISN'T THAT WHAT IT'S ALL ABOUT?

The following are some common stress-inducing thoughts for people of all ages. Find the statements that best pertain to you and re-think them into more positive thoughts. Challenge yourself and see if you can find a friend or family member who can benefit from the same or different ones. I'm sure you'll even think of people who could use this book, but it may not be in your best interest or the best time to ask them, so just enjoy a good laugh at the mere thought of the less-than-positive person who comes to mind.

Notice some of the stress-inducing language, like "hate," "always," and "never." These words not only make the negative thought more stressful than it needs to be, it also perpetuates it longer than it needs to be experienced. It is very important to isolate the stressful thought as soon as you notice it and change it to a healthier thought rather than, having it take over your overall mood and disposition for an extended period.

How can you "re-think" these thoughts and change your attitude about a person or the situation to reduce your stress level? A lot of these thoughts can be replaced by gratitude in a similar area. Take #1 for example, "I'm too tired to go to school (or work) today!" You could replace this thought with something like, "but I am grateful to receive an education (or have a job). Or, "but at least I'll earn money to pay my bills." Or, "I can nap later or go to bed earlier tonight."

What other negative attitudes/thoughts are you experiencing? (Fill in #99 and #100)

Think thoughts about our mental, physical, and/or spiritual health to help us feel our best! The more often you practice, the more it will become a habit, sooner than later.

If you feel negative and/or depressed
for an extended period of time, and
what you have tried or are currently
doing isn't helping, seek help
immediately.

1. **I'm too tired to go to school (or work) today!**

____

____

____

____

2. This weather sucks!

3. I hate being late!

4. I'm ugly!

____

____

____

____

____

5. My friends and I are having "issues!"

6. I'm so burnt out!

7. I hate my boss!

8. I hate my co-workers!

9. I don't
want to
be here in
this
moment!

10.

There's not enough time in the day!

11. Nobody understands me!

12. I hate slow drivers!

13. I'm fat!

14. S/he will never go out with me!

15. My kids/co-workers/ peers are driving me crazy!

16. I'm so sick of school!

17. I hate my job!

18. I have no money!

19. I'm bored!

20. I just can't get up since daylight savings time!

21. This fog/these clouds make me feel dreary!

22. I don't think I can do it!

23. It's Monday!

24. I don't like my mother- (or father) in-law

**25.
I don't like
my sibling's
significant
other!**

26. I don't like my brother (or sister)-in-law!

27. My in-laws don't like me!

28. I don't like my child's choices!

____

____

____

____

____

29.
**This event
is not like I
thought it
would be!**

____

____

____

____

____

30.
I am having problems with my significant other!

31.
I don't like grocery shopping!

32. I hate going to the mall!

33.
I am so uncoordinated!

34. I am not good at that!

35.
I don't feel like exercising!

36. I don't have enough time to get a good workout!

37. S/he's so stupid!

38. It's too hot!

39. It's too cold!

40. It's too early!

49

41. It's too late!

42.
I hate extra-curricular classes!

43. I hate math!

44. I hate science!

45. I hate social studies!

____

____

____

____

____

46. I hate reading!

47. I hate writing!

48. **My body hurts when I work out!**

49. I never have any clever ideas!

50. My nails are weak and brittle!

51. I don't have a green thumb!

52.

**I can't ski
or
snowboard!**

____

____

____

____

____

53. I don't have enough energy to get through the day!

54. I feel fat in these pants!

55.
I'm so disorganized!

56. I'm not a good worker!

57. I'm not a good co-worker!

____

____

____

____

____

58. I'm a lousy boss!

59.
I never know what to get people for a gift!

60. I don't have any talents!

61. I'm a
bad
friend!

62. I'm a bad sibling!

63. I'm too pale!

____

____

____

____

____

**64.
I never give
myself enough
time to self-
reflect for
improvement!**

65. I'm not worth it!

____

____

____

____

____

66.
I don't have
any
motivation!

67. I have bad body odor!

68.
The drive through messed up my order... AGAIN!

69.

**My allergies
are always
so bad in
the spring!**

**70. I could
never be
an
athlete
like you!**

71.
I spilled all the toothpicks all over the floor!

72.
I forgot our anniversary!

73.
I forgot my dad's birthday!

74.

I will never
be able to
get this
baby weight
off!

75.

I'm going to turn out to be like one of my relatives my family doesn't like!

76. I feel weird!

77.
I'm so different from everyone else!

78. I don't fit in!

79. I wish I had a specific electronic device or game system!

80. My car isn't cool!

81. I hate listening to people talking about politics!

82.

**I hate the
colors on my
walls in my
house but don't
have the money
to change
them!**

83. Same speed, same lane!

84.
I hate my neighbors!

85. I can't have children!

**86.
Nobody
understands
changes I've
made to feel
better about
myself!**

87.
I don't know which religion to be!

88. **I want to go back to school but can't afford it!**

89. I'm the worst parent!

90.
I feel
intimidated!

91.
I wish s/he would return my effort to reach out!

92. I don't know what to do!

93. I don't know what to say!

94. No diet works!

95.
I don't
know how
to improve
my
character!

96. **I want to go to that party but there will be people there I don't like!**

97. **The company that is providing a service for me isn't fair!**

98. I'll never heal from my injury!

99.

100.